MW00883124

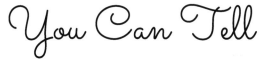

You Can Tell

Reflections from a medical educator

Written by Dr. Gabriel M. Aisenberg

ISBN-13: 978-1542350389
ISBN-10: 1542350387

ACKNOWLEDGEMENTS

The world may not belong to those who do more, but it certainly feels like that. Therefore, I thank my parents Gloria and José for teaching me to walk the extra mile.

I thank my stepfather Dr. Giora Cukier for showing me what I wanted to become and for succeeding at that.

Along the path, many doctors and patients modeled my actual self. I want to highlight the influence of Dr. Herbert Fred's, a mentor and a friend, to whom I owe not only a good part of my knowledge but most of my wisdom.

Finally, I would not be who I am without the love, support, and encouragement of my family: my wife Cynthia, whose eyes always find the best in everyone, even me, and my children Lucas, Tomás, and Carola. You make everything worthwhile.

INDEX

PROLOGUE

The time for reflection upon our practice is scarce, particularly out of the academic environment. Resulting from this scarcity, there is a sensation of automatism overlying our encounters with patients, colleagues, and ancillary services. In this setting, finding meaning to our actions as doctors results troublesome.

This collection of reflections was born when I was a fellow of the Health Educator Program at the University of Texas in Houston. The mandate was to collect twelve of them, and they would represent "phrases, skills, or tools that helped our academic experiences."

As I kept practicing as an Internal Medicine attending at Lyndon Baines Johnson Hospital, I realized that certain problems tended to appear more often, making certain educational interventions (lectures, articles, mine and others', advice, and thoughts) more frequent than others. This made the accrual of the "needed twelve" very easy. More importantly, it created in me a mindset where reflection is a must, and documenting and sharing what I learned, another educational opportunity.

This book is based on almost thirty years of practice, and invites the reader to generate his or her own reflective diary. In the end, it is the path we walk that teaches us.

Gabriel Aisenberg, MD, FACP

Chapter 1
PATIENT AT THE CENTER

1

Doctors are powerful people. Our power lies in our words. When we speak, people listen to us. Therefore we need to make sure that our advice is arising from, and backed up by the right source of information. "With great power comes great responsibility."

Feb 4, 2012

2

Each clinical encounter is like a movie already started. You are surrounded by darkness, and in front of you a scene depicts a situation you are yet to understand. However, unlike the movie, our intervention can lead the path to a happy ending.

Apr 1, 2012

3

There are four reasons to order a test: the right one and three wrong ones: fear of litigation, plain ignorance, and reimbursement. The latter predominates in the private world (although the other two may still be present).

The academic world is in most places the only way to deal with the above issues, by teaching the learners the benefit of teaching the patients what is the right way to go, the benefit of time and patience observing the natural evolution of diseases, the possibility to divert from the original plan, and the reassuring presence of the doctor at the side of his/her patients. The best way to avoid being defensive doctors is being real doctors.

Aug 25, 2012

4

When you offer your patient a diagnostic or therapeutic intervention, ask them to ask you four questions:

What happen if I don't do it? That is, the natural evolution of the disease.

What good things are expected from doing it? The benefit expected from the intervention.

What bad things are expected from doing it? The side effects, adverse in general.

What are the alternatives?

Empowering the patient is the goal. We want the patients to feel that they are playing a card game, but not only knowing their own cards, but the opponent's too. There is no way to lose.

Oct 26, 2012

5

For those who believe in fate: I was on the verge of becoming absolutely arrogant, when a piece of advice from the unexpected character led me back to the righteous path. My grandfather was fighting advanced colon cancer a few months prior to my wedding. In those days I was an intern. Urged to have him by my side during *my* moment, and believing that science can cure it all, I was by his hospital bedside telling him to get better so he could come to my wedding. His answer was short (of breath and of words): "You, doctors, don't understand us patients."

I have spent more than a quarter century honoring him, doing my best to understand those I care for.

April 26, 2015

6

On house calls:

The history we get from our patients represents in most cases the subjective experience of their own lives, their own perception. It's not that they lie to us (sometimes they do); it's that they just fail to recognize the influence of their environment and actions over their actual selves. A short visit to our patients' homes will teach us about how they live, what every day anguishes and limitations affect their lives, what usually mild changes in their behavior and surroundings may deeply affect their outcomes. Even if there is no payment, there is certainly a reward.

April 26, 2015

7

I usually tell my ward learners "At the end of this rotation I want at least one person to hate you, and try that person not to be me." Sometimes the price of efficacy in the care of one's patients is to make other people do their job. From the distance, the nagging learner will be the patient's hero, but often will look to others like an arrogant or braggart. I believe that this is a price worth paying.

May 4, 2015

8

The patient makes a statement about his own belief on the disease that ails him.

I'd never heard of the association he mentions, but instead of closing the door, I go ahead and read.

It turns out that the association has not been described the way he presents, but there are some similarities in shape, but not time: the patient's picture is chronic and the described association is acute.

The end of the day comes; what did I learn? That I still don't know what my patient has. That maybe I just discovered a potential explanation for his condition, though it has not been documented in the literature. That maybe the next case in which the association appears will make my case stronger.

I reflect on all this and conclude that curiosity fuels the engine of science; that everything was discovered for the first time at some point; that, especially for the complicated cases, it is better to keep our minds open.

Aug 6, 2015

9

Today someone died. A patient. I barely knew her for she came to me on the same day. Everywhere, everyone was foreseeing this moment. The family was around. There was a husband, two adult children, another woman the patient's generation. Everyone cried. For them it's not just another life gone. For them it is the sum of all the good and bad memories. The certainty of a future without their loved one. We offer our sympathy that is only sincere when we reflect on our empathy. Today, I lost someone...

Aug 6, 2015

10

Most of us agree on what harming a patient is, and how important it is not to do so. The principle of non-maleficence is without a doubt the most relevant guide for our practice. But not everyone agrees on what is good for a patient. The moral obligation to help patients with terminal diseases (ruled by the principle of beneficence) is limited by the patient's desire to accept invasive interventions (ruled by the principle of autonomy), the coexistence of multiple serious symptoms that curtail the improvement expected from treating them individually, the costs associated with the intervention, as well as its availability (ruled by the principle of justice), and the always uncertain life expectancy.

Feb 28, 2016

11

If you want your patient to fast, don't just enter an order; tell your patient.

If you want your patient to eat, don't just enter an order; tell your patient.

If you want your patient to take a medication, don't just enter an order; tell your patient.

If you want your patient to give blood for a test, or to get some imaging study, don't just enter an order; tell your patient.

The patient is at the center of what we do, and even if his or her educational level is below the one needed to understand complex explanation, it is our duty to make it simple.

Mar 20, 2016

12

Be there for your patient. Currently the healthcare system is so compartmentalized that no one knows who the patient's doctor is: neither the multiple involved providers nor the patient. A simple gesture; giving your patients your pager or cell phone number will represent a soothing anxiety therapy. Analyze even this practical reason: it's better to get your patients' call than their lawyer's.

Mar 20, 2016

13

As much as I care for people, I cannot tell anyone to get sick to understand patients. However, there is a lot to learn from feeling sick. When we feel sick it is hard to keep interested in assisting others. It is difficult to collect the energy to help others; our senses get blunted, and with that the diagnostic skills. Otherwise pleasurable experiences stopped being so. Advice to the younger minds: stay healthy if you want to keep helping.

Dec 4, 2016

14

Two relevant aspects of patient care arise from the right diagnosis: the treatment (when available or possible) and the prognosis. Therefore, we should make every possible step towards finding the right diagnosis, ideally avoiding the contaminated version of it resulting from unnecessary, often misleading tests and from therapies that, in most cases, can wait.

Dec 4, 2016

15

The battle against death is lost, and since we all have to go, it is our duty to analyze in detail the process of dying, to make sure we help our patients until the end.

Most doctors will agree that the most important vital organ is the brain; and when the brain stops working, hope of recovery usually stops with it. Before that happens, the next two vital organs in order of importance, the heart and the lungs, usually stop. We call that cardiopulmonary arrest.

The essence of this story lies exactly in understanding that lungs and heart usually stop working after battling disease that does not have a treatment, or was treated but failed to get over ailment. Proportionally, just a few cases of cardiopulmonary arrest occur as a result of acute, reversible processes (cardiac arrhythmia, a blocked coronary artery, electrolyte anomalies, and some more).

When we ask our patients whether they want us, "almighty doctors," to bring the function of those organs back, we tend to do so in a concrete, decontextualized setting, offering a menu of two options: yes and no. I believe our duty to be more paternalistic. The experienced doctor knows that the maneuvers employed to resuscitate heart, lungs and brain are seldom successful, at least in terms of leaving a patient able to function afterwards. If such actions only lead to the same circumstances that just made the heart and lungs stop, and the underlying disease has no chance to improve, the resuscitative efforts are not only futile, but also harmful.

Not every death is the same. A careful, patient-centered explanation usually helps doing what is right.

Dec 20, 2016

16

The doctor at his patient's funeral. Once again, death won the battle. The corpse is exhibited in a wooden coffin. Here, and there, people cry. Others laugh nervously to escape their own anxiety, the fear of the inevitable. A few more attentive attendees look at the doctor. Could he have done some more? Could he have delayed this moment? Why does the patient's son embrace this man, whose efforts were unsuccessful? Were those efforts enough? And what is the meaning of that silence between them, so loaded with body language, with tears, with emotion?

Many experiences enrich us as doctors. Attending our patients' funerals is our final duty and sign of respect for those that are no longer strangers. They were generous to include us in their stories; we must now celebrate their lives.

Dec 20, 2016

Chapter 2
KNOWLEDGE IS RELATIVE

17

Sometimes when I have troubles figuring out how to solve a problem, I push myself to the thought of the only certainty of my own existence (*Cogito, ergo sum*). Then, as if nothing else was invented, I try to put together flexible, ever-changing pieces to build the puzzle that will bring the answer.

In patient care, the names of those pieces are knowledge, skills, law, ethics, empathy, and spirituality (or religion).

Mar 9, 2012

18

Knowing is not everything in medicine.

Caring is more important than knowing. Caring fuels our days to go that necessary extra mile never noticed by virtually anyone. Caring drives our curiosity; it motivates the questions that lead to the solutions to our patients' problems. Caring changes our priorities, putting the patient first, or the learners first when our main activity is teaching. It's not too different from parenting.

Understanding is more important than knowing. Understanding is energy-saving. A few bits of information are needed, and then it's all about making the connections, letting A lead to B, and so on.

Knowledge acquisition requires the other two. But it also demands self-discipline, time, access to material to acquire knowledge from, and the guidance of someone more expert to get it right.

I know it...

Jan 17, 2014

19

Skepticism is a must, but it should not result simply from stubbornness. When a patient tells us something, it is our obligation to see the consistency in those words, the likelihood for that to be a fair statement. But beware of the doctors that amplify that information and are fast to label patients with conditions they may not have. Furthermore, always remember that not all that is written in an electronic medical record is true.

Feb 28, 2016

20

Knowledge is sexy. Knowledge is power. But, knowledge is also volatile. What is known today becomes history in a blink, for there is virtually no axiom in medicine. New philosophy adds to the old ones, but new science replaces the old one.

Mar 1, 2016

21

I am careful to be harsh on my learners' knowledge. At any given moment they may know -at least about something- more than I do. The purpose of a syllabus is to determine what the minimum grasp of a broad content must be, but in truth, learning never ends. Unfortunately, the whole body of knowledge -that is, everything that is to be known- grows exponentially, while the individual can only learn at an arithmetic speed. The sad consequence is that relatively speaking, we know less and less every minute.

Mar 1, 2016

22

Knowledge creates bias. Every time we see a patient we ask questions based on what we know. Unfortunately, at any given time what we don't know is way more than what we do know. Therefore, there will always be questions not asked, and others that will provide us with useless information. We must always keep our minds open.

Jul 2, 2016

23

Let us eat garbage. Two billion flies can't be mistaken.
Remain cautious when the explanation that backs up your colleagues' actions is nothing but "this is what most doctors would do."

Dec 20, 2016

24

On risk factors:

The majority of what we call risk factors for multiple diseases is known to us by looking back in the lives of patients with those diseases, and comparing the presence of the presumed cause in that group of patients, with that one in a corresponding group of people just without the disease at stake. We call that the odds ratio.

Being that under usual circumstances the state of health is more common than the absence of it, using the above strategy misses a relevant point. Many people, the majority in fact, of those with the disease may not have the studied risk factor, and a considerable number of healthy people (at least as far as the studied disease is concerned) may carry the scrutinized risk factor. When we assume that the higher proportion in which the risk factor presents among the ill compared to the sane is enough proof for that factor to be the cause of the disease, we expose ourselves to being misled and biased.

The untrained mind may assume that someone's chest pain represents a heart attack when that person has close relatives with coronary atherosclerosis, and personal exposure to smoking, to uncontrolled diabetes mellitus, high blood pressure and every known "'risk factor' under the sun, even when blood is leaking from the wound caused by a knife still sticking in that person's chest.

Innumerable fallacies have been accrued throughout the history of medicine. We shall remember that statistics offer us a tool, but occasionally we run into significant data (from a mathematical perspective) with little if any biological plausibility. If you care for your patient, allow your skeptical mind to keep connecting the dots, regardless of what others observed, and challenge everyone if you disagree.

Dec 20, 2016

25

On consults:

Consultants often have one or a few more diplomas hanging from their walls. Those pieces of paper only tell the world that the colleagues have spent longer time studying a fraction of what's there to be learned, specializing in a more restricted content.
When you call a consultant, make sure you know what you want to learn from him or her. The question must be pertinent to the case. You must have read about the patient's condition and elevated the level of sophistication of your query, in order to make evident that the only difference between you and your consultant –at least when it comes to the issue at stake- is an expectedly larger experience on the specialist's side.

Dec 20, 2016

26

Learn to break the mold. Guidelines are crutches; only those that cannot walk would use them. Even if most people would act in a certain way when facing your patient's problem, you are still your patient's best advocate. Therefore, acknowledge what you don't know, recognize the individuality of your patient's case, look for someone more experienced than you, read until your eyes itch. Only then you are ready to make a decision for your patient.

Dec 20, 2016

Chapter 3
COST, PRICE, AND VALUE

27

Think broad, act narrow. Many things potentially explain the phenomena in front of our eyes. In most scenarios, it is enough to use our deductive skills to determine the main problem and act upon it. In most of those times, the exclusion of the alternative explanations (or diagnoses) is just a matter of an extra mental effort, rather than expensive, and many times unnecessary, diagnostic tests.

Jun 18, 2012

28

What will be left when our diagnostic skills, when our doctor-patient communication, when our physical exams, are no longer needed? What will be of medicine when for a few quarters people go somewhere to get a (presumably) harmless pan-scan that will spit up many diagnoses, and, why not, many therapeutic suggestions?

I believe I know the answer: medicine will be boring. I still wonder if this option will be beneficial for patients. It will if it brings further questions that require further interpretation (maybe the only leftover role for doctors in this utopian scenario). Very likely, such sensitive "super-diagnostic-machine" will fail to rule out the false positives.

Jul 19, 2012

29

In one occasion a resident was taking care of a man whose creatinine level was three times the one at baseline. The patient said he had been vomiting for a few days, while still taking diuretics, treating his underlying heart failure. The cause for the acute renal dysfunction seemed evident. Yet, the resident wanted to make sure that there was not an obstructive cause. I decided to create the following challenge: from that moment on, if someone wanted to order a test that could have waited until we proved failure to respond to treatment of the most likely cause, and the performed test added no diagnostic or management value, then the resident would owe me the price of that test (with the added benefit of learning such price). I was so sure of this approach that I would tell the residents that I'd pay twice that price back if the seemingly unneeded test did yield a management-changing result.

I keep collecting money…

May 15, 2015

30

The electronic medical record certainly corrects problems related to the infamous doctors' handwriting, and it has become in itself a teaching tool when it comes to picking -at least in certain circumstances- the right dose of certain medications. However, some concerns arise in the following circumstances:

a- When doctors learn the opinion of their consultants from a written note, rather than from talking to them. I know as a fact that no note reflects a hundred percent of anyone's opinion (at least that is the case for my notes); therefore, asking for an opinion to a colleague, even if it's just his or her gut feeling, gives me (and the colleague) the reassuring sensation of being on the same page, plus the benefit for both of us that we know we care. Even as a business model, the call may represent an invitation for a future interaction with that particular colleague.

b- Putting an order doesn't make it happen. Not all the diagnostic tests are adequately represented in the system, and our mistakes can lead to a paralyzing confusion. Talking to the laboratory, the radiologist, or the pharmacy tends to overcome this problem.

c- Removing an order doesn't make it stop. I witnessed many unnecessary tests done in spite of the formal removal of the order, simply because the provider (that being MRI, CT scan, or certain consults) was not called on time, or the patient was not empowered in that direction. This needs not to be complex. Examples include orders for fasting not complied by the patients because they simply don't know the order was there. The same is valid for monitoring the urinary output or daily weights.

That subject made of flesh, blood, and bone keeps (or must so) being at the center of our activities.

Feb 28, 2016

31

What difference does it make to offer health insurance to everyone, if the service is focused on making money or defensive medicine? In the current situation, the government is promoting access to affordable (at least more than before) healthcare for part of the 30% of uninsured patients in exchange for tax benefits. The logical and laudable intention is that people now access early diagnoses to avoid secondary morbidity and mortality. When healthcare providers see now more patients with these plans, there is at least a chance that an excess of studies will happen, not following general age-based recommendations, but prejudice: "because these patients were never studied before, and we don't know how long they will remain insured, order every possible diagnostic test now; if they generate reimbursement for the clinic, even better." In fact, I encountered patients that told me to "order everything, for I have insurance now." Unfortunately, writing an order takes a tenth of the time needed to explain why those studies are not needed.

Dec 4, 2016

32

We must wonder: is access to healthcare a right or a privilege? The way things are set, only the accommodated classes in the United States access fast and good quality and quantity of services. For the middle class, these services might still be available, but since the consequence of cost reduction is usually higher deductibles and copays, patients elect not to go to the doctor, aware of the possible oncoming expenses. The poor are always the poor: in absence of a safety net, they only access healthcare when they feel too sick, and this usually represents irreversible bodily damage, foreboding nothing but the inability to work, and therefore, to pay for future healthcare needs.

In a system based on solidarity, a proportional, income-based payment of a national or state health insurance would warrant access to healthcare for everyone. Being that the cost of services is high, many times overpriced, this approach carries the risk of stratifying the available resources to assure basic services for everyone, while the most expensive ones would be delivered on a first-come-first-served basis, or, following the American style, allowing extra money to access faster care.

The way I see it, the product of the healthcare factory is the healthy worker, who, being healthy, works, earns a salary, pays taxes, and contributes his or her part to the health insurance. Only such equalitarian system would warrant healthcare being a right.

Dec 4, 2016

33

Most of the patients coming to the hospital do so through the Emergency Center (EC). This area is usually responsible for close to 70% of admissions to general hospitals. It was not until the early 1970's that the EC was assigned to Emergency physicians and mid-level providers of the same specialty. Until then, the care for patients suffering emergent medical conditions was directed by clinicians, surgeons, or obstetricians, depending on the diagnosis. Nowadays, the status of the American healthcare system overemphasizes the role and practice of the EC. This is in part because the EC is obliged by federal law to care for the patients suffering from emergent conditions. However, many patients define emergencies differently than the medical dictionary does, therefore making the trip to the place that needs no appointment while providing with a one-time stop for studies to assess their conditions. Moreover, the health insurances blindly pay for the expenses, because the patients' conditions are defined as emergent. There is no defense against this perverse system. The focus of "pay-for-performance" strategies is on verifying that certain conditions (pneumonia, myocardial infarction, and ischemic stroke) are treated in a timely and standardized way, but pays no attention to the excess of studies or treatment for those diseases, or to the care of less incident conditions. The way I see it, if a hammer only recognizes nails, the EC caregiver will only see emergencies. The care for the non-emergent patient in the EC must be transferred to doctors that have the patience and knowledge to care for them in a timely, patient-centered, and cost-effective way.

Dec 4, 2016

Chapter 4
MEDICAL EDUCATION

34

The learning process has become too passive. Learners are always looking up to their teachers for information rather than for advice.

In order for the learners to be active characters in their own growing process, they need not to be spoon-fed with answers, but to know that they are accountable for their progress, empowered to that duty, allowing them to know that the expectations upon them are high.

One idea is to ask the learners what they would do if they led the team, if they were to make decisions.

Nov 22, 2011

35

I remember the days of my first residency in Buenos Aires (1990-1993). We didn't have a hospital library. To pick up an article I had to get on a bus, travel for 20 minutes, review the "Index Medicus" (each volume a 2-inch wide book with only one month of literature citations), select the articles, pray for the journals to be part of the library collection, ask the librarian for the copies, and return 2 days later to pick them up.

Nowadays, with remote access to thousands of journals, the answers are easy to reach.

Therefore, where there is a doubt, there should be an answer. And where there is no answer, there is an opportunity for research.

Dec 10, 2011

36

Communication and leadership represent the basis for a successful team. When holding themselves accountable, and keeping no secrets from the other team members (at least when it comes to team-related matters), even the unlikely victors are able to succeed.

In that setting, leadership is needed to help solve problems and to give tools to other team members to reach their highest level. Unlike other types of teams, teaching-medical teams usually have short-term goals and a fast turnover of their focus (new patients every day). Still, the basic rules above apply.

Apr 15, 2012

37

We can teach a lot on "how to teach" but how can we measure the outcome? Is our trainees' performance enough? Or does that tell us more about them than about us? Are the teaching awards any better or more representative than the monthly evaluations by our trainees? Where does the subjectivity of a peer evaluation finish? And how about the objectivity of case managers, nurses, patients?

May 2, 2012

38

No patient will teach us better that the one on whom doing nothing is the best we can do. The natural evolution of a disease has multiple presentations, but determining features of severity is generally easy to do. For those on whom the diagnosis is unclear, and when features of severity are not present, consider waiting as your best intervention. Particularly in the hospital setting, changing your mind at the right time is still likely to help your patient, and not needing to do so gives you the unique chance of understanding that many times our patients improve in spite of what we do, rather than because of what we do.

Oct 27, 2012

39

I tell my students, "I'm not better than you; just older. I am not here to teach you what, but how. I certainly don't own the truth, but perhaps that doesn't matter; for what it is considered truth today may not be so tomorrow."

This, for a young mind still trying to find its shape, may be paralyzing. Yet, it is amazing -at least to me- to see that moment in which the students develop the germ of skepticism, and instead of giving up, they get the energy to start looking for that metaphor of the truth that we call evidence.

I thank the graduating class for learning so much from what they don't know, and the school for allowing me to promote that technique.

Apr 5, 2014 (for McGovern Award 2014)

40

The dawn of every doctor's relationship with knowledge is chaotic, as if what is to be known belonged in a different dimension. Aware of his own ignorance, the future academician must *learn how to learn*, how to connect the innumerable dots in the otherwise disorganized universe surrounding him.

As time elapses, the doctor becomes a doctor, and then, the moment to give back emerges. Now it is time to *learn how to teach*, to develop the techniques necessary to share with others the tools to organize the ever growing fund of knowledge.

The learner inherits from the teacher the tools to make the transmission of knowledge not only more efficient, but also more focused and determined; the goal is now to nurture the next generation of doctors. The teacher *teaches how to learn*.

Finally, some of the members of this new generation will be driven by the desire of restarting the circle; the older generation will *teach how to teach*, and then complete the academic cycle. New teachers are being born.

I believe that academic physicians should be aware of their own limited ability to know facts and of the frailty of what we call evidence, for this evidence changes at a fast pace, forcing our minds and attitude to adapt. Scientific skepticism is the best tool to abide by this concept. Always challenge the current version of the truth: if after scrutiny the concept being challenged survives, then it becomes reliable; if it doesn't, then new evidence replaces the old one.

Jun 9, 2014

GOALS FOR THE WARD MONTH:

1-Be happy: if you are not happy, you can't help others.

2-Be curious: the only way to fill a gap in your knowledge is to discover that you have such a gap. Review the disease process of each one of your patients, and make sure that you understood what your patient has and what the plan is. Ask your upper-level or your attending. Don't be shy.

3-Be generous: share what you've learned with your teammates. Send the evidence behind your learning issues to everyone within the team.

4-Be outspoken, but respectful: you are part of a team, and as inexpert as you can be, your opinion counts.

5-Imagine you are the attending: feel with your gut that the patient is *yours*. I truly enjoy when I see the patients relate to you as if you were the boss. Nevertheless, let the patient know what your role is.

6-Whatever your role is, from now on KEEP UP WITH THE RESIDENT SPIRIT. Don't ever give up the process. It will increase your level of satisfaction and the efficiency with which you help others.

7-At the end of every day, make sure you reflect upon the experiences you lived that day. Discover the meaning, not only the evidence.

Some time in 2010, but posted on April 26, 2015

42

When I evaluate a student or a resident, there must be a core group of objective features that should at least match expectations. Still a fraction of my comments, probably more related to art and style, will be subjective. For the latter, my scope would be based on the likelihood of that learner of becoming my doctor.

April 29, 2015

43

There are two aspects of medicine not adequately taught: pathophysiology and the natural history of any given disease.

I am not certain of the reasons for the former. However, I cannot but emphasize the importance of such teaching. Physiology is the study of the bodily functions, at a global level, at a system level, at an organ level, and at a cellular level. Understanding how a cell, tissue, organ, system, or the body normally function, make easy understanding how they don't. The study of such dysfunction is called pathophysiology. The phenotypic presentation of such dysfunctions, that is signs and symptoms of disease, is the subject of study of Internal Medicine.

I understand better why we don't teach well the natural history of any given disease. To start, only if we are diligent, or lucky, or both, we can understand the origin of the signs and symptoms of the disease before the current presentation. The problem is rather that we will not wait to see the course of the disease for too long, either because we are too prone to intervene (to treat) even before we know the diagnosis, or too prone to send people their way before we are certain of their outcome. This is in time explained by financial pressures or self-imposed needs to decrease the hospital census.

May 4, 2015

44

Case reports and case series suit the generalist academicians' need to promote the advancement of science. Being that, as Dr. Herbert Fred says, "All patients are interesting, but not all doctors are interested," case reports provide the interested physicians with the opportunity to straightforwardly take the case, or at least some aspect of it, to a higher level of understanding. This tool is versatile, for it allows documentation of the common presentation of uncommon diseases, uncommon presentation of common diseases, peculiarities of patient management (even when encountered by chance), and sets the stage for future research by promoting the development of new questions. Even if the manuscript does not get published, the review of the literature required to support the case carries an educational value.

Mar 1, 2016

45

Medical schools need researchers: the scientists whose ideas represent the germ of the medicine of tomorrow. But they also need academicians, that is, teachers. Most medical schools are ranked today upon the monies that support their research. In the context, generalists who prefer to keep their focus of research all encompassing, rather than centered on specific topics have fewer opportunities to fund that vital activity. This, in turn, creates several problems. The largest funding institutions consider the researcher's expertise when allocating their grants. Therefore, a clinician with questions pertaining to too many disciplines pays the price of his curiosity by decreasing the chance of being awarded with funds. Furthermore, most of the scattered resources are placed on funding randomized trials, set at the top of the evidence pyramid. Prospective research is then a virtually impossible task. To complete this vicious cycle, younger investigators will more likely prefer to join senior physicians with narrow expertise, increasing their own chances of being funded.

Mar 1, 2016

46

Here we go again. A new academic year starts. New faces, younger-appearing than the ones I saw last year, get ready to present the story of patients extremely complex -as simple as they might be- for their skills. They fear me and my every day older look; they fear their residents, barely more experienced than them; and more importantly, they fear their own ignorance. The real deal just started, and they have to "become doctors in no time." Beyond the frustration that this situation brings, these are the times that separate the good from the great teachers.

Jul 2, 2016

47

No words are more influential for the actions of the curious doctor (or learner) than "I don't know." Naturally, the more we grow in our profession, the more likely we know more answers. But as importantly, our confidence grows too and what we don't know becomes an invitation to do something about it: read, ask someone else... The good doctor (or learner) will accept that invitation while acknowledging loudly what remains unknown.

Sep 11, 2016

48

Look for sources of wisdom beyond the patient's bedside. Culture (all that is not nature) adopts different forms: music, painting, sculpture, movies, literature... Wise creators of quotable phrases can be found everywhere. From these fountains of knowledge, we can see and use what we like and dislike, and we can emphasize (medical) concepts to make them memorable. In short, culture is the part of life that makes us the persons we need to be to help our patients.

Sep 11, 2016

49

One of our duties on patient care is to be aware of the constant threatening presence of the possibility of making a mistake, so we can strengthen our confidence as we search for the truth.

Dec 1, 2016

50

The way we think is influenced by previously acquired knowledge. Unless we make our curiosity prevail, the chance of being led (or misled) by what we know is high. Patients have what they have and not what we want them to have. Therefore, we should remove ourselves from a position of certainty, labeling a patient with a diagnosis, and instead collect the data, recognize a problem, and establish the diagnosis for each patient we see.

Dec 4, 2016

Made in the USA
San Bernardino, CA
20 March 2017